My

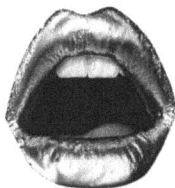

My!

My

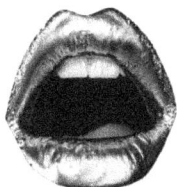

My!

A Committed Woman's Guide to
Getting the *Great Sex* She Deserves

Brandye Wilson-Manigat, MD

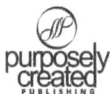

purposely
created
PUBLISHING

MY O MY!
Published by Purposely Created Publishing Group™
Copyright © 2020 Brandye Wilson-Manigat
All rights reserved.

Printed in the United States of America

ISBN: 978-1-64484-185-3

Special discounts are available on bulk quantity purchases by book clubs, associations and special interest groups. For details email: sales@publishyourgift.com or call (888) 949-6228.
For information log on to www.PublishYourGift.com

*This book is dedicated to my mother
for supporting me and teaching me courage
in the face of adversity.*

TABLE OF CONTENTS

INTRODUCTION

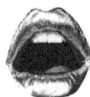

Iwrote this book to tell the truth about sex and orgasm for women and to create a safe space for women to learn about how their bodies work. One of my passions is in dispelling myths and misinformation and empowering women to have conversations about taboo subjects while becoming masters of their bodies and sexual experiences. But not only that, my goal is to teach women how to make feeling good their default. I wrote this book because this is what I wish I had many years ago when I needed all of this information in one place. I wrote this book for the teenage me who would check out books about sex at the library because I wanted to understand it. Even at that time, I knew there was more to sex than "insert tab A into slot B."

We do a disservice to society when women are left in the dark about how their bodies work and what their true capabilities are. Women succumb to the myth that pleasure is only for their partner and not for them. They carry the limiting belief that something is inherently wrong with them, and this shows up not only in the bedroom but also in their performance at work, their child-rearing, and their interactions with other women. Women are constantly comparing themselves to other women instead of standing in the power of who they are. The world needs women to step into their power, show up fully, and unleash their feminine essence into the world.

Education has always been important to me and my family. I grew up in a single-parent home in South Central Los Angeles, and my mom always impressed upon me the importance of education for getting ahead in life. But I had dreams of doing more. From the age of 10, I dreamed of becoming a doctor. I was the first in my family to graduate college, and I went on to study medicine at UCLA and become a physician. I purposely decided on Women's Health and Obstetrics and Gynecology because it was an opportunity to educate and empower women as well as influence the health of entire families. And when I was done with residency, I embarked on starting my own private practice desiring to continue helping women have their best health overall. However, having the private practice took a toll on my own health and well-being including my marriage. I was overwhelmed and not interested in anything but sleeping. And to go along with that, my sex life and marriage were suffering. I tried all of the quick fixes, lingerie, *50 Shades of Grey*, and toys, but none of it lasted. Nothing made any long-term difference. I was afraid that I was broken. I was afraid that I'd lost my sexy and would never get it back. I was afraid that I was going to lose my husband. So, I set out on a mission to change my life! I found out that sex was more than just a physical act and that the lack of it was a sign of something deeper. I healed my bedroom story. And as I went along that journey, I began meeting women who were also struggling in this area. It was the highlight of my day to educate and empower them to get their sexy back. And I have been on a crusade ever since to teach women how to feel good in and out of the bedroom.

CHAPTER 1

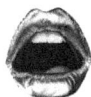

WHAT'S GOING ON
WITH YOUR SEXY?

In the beginning you couldn't keep your hands off of each other. You hugged, cuddled, kissed and loved on each other all the time. Life was good! Then...your life got complicated. You both progressed in your careers, racking up titles and responsibilities. You started a family. You began living the American dream. And now your time is filled with running kids to school, coordinating who is picking them up and dropping them off for after school activities, wiping sticky hands and faces, and helping with homework and science projects that are due the next day! There are no more lingering hugs and holding hands. You barely look each other in the eyes to say hello. You don't smile at each other. You are on the battlefield, and gone are the niceties. Instead, your time is spent putting out fires and trying to stick to the daily routine. You know, that performance you do every day to make sure all the plates keep spinning and that none of them falls and breaks. And once you both fall into bed, you hope your partner goes to sleep quickly and doesn't reach for you because you just don't have the energy or the desire for sex. You still love him. He's a great husband, father, and provider. But when he asks you why you can't have sex tonight, all you've got for him is "I'm tired" or "I have to get up early for work tomorrow." And you feel justified in your reasons because *"Damn it, you are working your ass off every day."* But in those rare alone moments when you are reflecting on your life, you think, "Is this all there is to my life?"

You are not alone. So many women are living lives of quiet desperation, trying to be Superwoman. We are trying to be great at work, an awesome mom, a helpful daughter, and an amazing wife ready to please her partner. The actual statistics for the number of women struggling with low or no interest in sex is not known. Why is this? Well, for one, few women are speaking up about it to anyone other than to their close female relatives or good girlfriends. Secondly, few people are asking questions about women's sexual desire and lack thereof. Thirdly, up until recently, there was no incentive, monetary or otherwise, to create a magic bullet to solve the problem. So, women are suffering in silence with something they think has no solution. They believe this is just what happens with time. You get tired or bored and sleep just sounds more enticing than sex. You believe that as you age your sex drive is supposed to decline, and in the back of your head, you're thinking about making an appointment to see your doctor because *this must be menopause*.

Well, I have a newsflash for you: This is NOT menopause! Although a pause of a different sort has occurred. The ups and downs of life have combined to pause your connection and awareness of yourself and what you desire. It is like everyone else is more important than you, and (excuse the expression) they cum before you. You have given so much of yourself to everyone else that when it's time to even consider your own pleasure and sexual desire, you only see it as draining your already empty cup. But sex was never meant to come as an afterthought to your hectic, overwhelming schedule. Sex is a necessity for your overall health, well-being, and vitality. There is an energetic force tied to sex. It powers your confidence, creativity, and connection. And when that energy is blocked, it can put certain aspects of you in a dormant or sleep state.

There are some changes that happen to you, physically and otherwise, if you are not having sex regularly. There is a component of *use it or lose it*. If you are not thinking about it or doing it, this further suppresses any sexual thoughts or actions. Lack of sex can make relationships more vulnerable to anger, feelings of detachment and isolation, resentment, and bitterness that can build up and lead to infidelity and possibly divorce. Your intimate relationships are not the only ones that can suffer. Your lack of sex can show up as you become crankier, more critical, and irritable with your co-workers or your children. In addition, if you have not had sex in a while, it can make sex more difficult physically. It may be harder to have enough lubrication or for the vaginal tissues to comfortably stretch. These effects can be exacerbated by the hormonal changes that happen in menopause and perimenopause.

Besides ameliorating the physical changes that occur with the vaginal tissues, there are many other benefits to getting your sexy back. You become more awake to the world around you. If you've ever seen the movie, "The Wizard of Oz," it gives a good visual for how life is experienced with no or bad sex versus good sex. The movie starts off with the main character, Dorothy in Kansas. This part of the movie is in black and white. There is a tornado that lifts her house and carries her to the land of Oz. When the house lands, she is transported to a world that is in Technicolor. As Dorothy travels to the wizard to find a way back home, she learns so much about herself, her courage, her heart, and her inner wisdom. When you are having good sex, you see the world in Technicolor. You feel alive! You are able to learn more about yourself, your power and courage, your heart, and your inner wisdom.

Aside from getting to know yourself a bit better, here are a few other side effects of good sex. You are generally calmer and more relaxed. You feel more confident. Your blood pressure is usually lower, you sleep better, and you have less irritability and mood changes. Your intimate relationships generally improve. You have less pain. So, now you can't use that old standby, "Not tonight honey; I have a headache" because good sex and orgasm are an alternative to taking a pain pill.

Notes

Notes

Notes

Notes

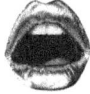

CHAPTER 2

WHAT IS GOOD SEX?

So, if you are having sex, wouldn't you like to have good sex? Otherwise, what's the point? Bad sex only makes things harder. If it is bad sex, you try to avoid it at all cost. You dread it and think of it as another task you should check off your to-do list instead of as a time for your pleasure and connection. *What do you want your sex life to be?* Do you want to keep dodging your partner, feeling like a bad partner, or feeling guilty because you know you should want sex? Do you want the same old boring routine to go on for the rest of your life because you are not willing to have the conversation with your partner about how his approach for sex could use a little work? *What do you want your sex life to look like?*

Sex was not meant to be a form of torture. Sex is an emotion in motion. It was meant to be a physical expression of the mental, emotional, and spiritual connections we have with ourselves and share with another person.

Before we start to outline the components necessary for good sex, I have to get on my soapbox for a few minutes. Sex is a gift from God for our benefit, not something that He is keeping from us. He created our brains and bodies to have those things necessary for pleasure. He is a good God!

Sex is not bad; it is sacred. The sacredness of sex is represented by the ultimate connection between two people, the union of two souls. It is not a frivolous decision to share your soul with another person. Before you do, know who you are sharing it with and wait and see who they are. You cannot know the true nature of a person from a few dates. Attraction can be fleeting and is not the basis for a solid relationship. My suggestion is before you begin an intimate relationship, make sure you have an intimate relationship with God and with yourself. This foundation will prepare you to be able to discern who is worthy to share your body and soul. This is the key to experiencing the sacredness of sex.

Whether you agree that sex should be reserved for marriage or are of the belief that religion has no place in the bedroom, I'm sure you want to have the best experience possible. Okay, I'm stepping down from my soapbox.

Good sex starts with good communication. You should discuss your likes and dislikes, boundaries, and absolute deal-breakers. During sex, communication is often nonverbal. Your sounds and face or body movements can communicate your level of pleasure and engagement. Communication after sex is also important. Most of the time, this can be something as simple as telling your partner, "That was great!" or just cuddling together.

Another important component of good sex is intimacy. Intimacy is defined as a close, familiar, and usually affectionate or loving, personal relationship with another person (Dictionary.com). Intimacy can be generated by simple things like holding hands while riding in the car together, providing your undivided attention while your partner is talking, buying a thoughtful gift, sending a "just thinking about you" text, or long, lingering hugs.

Sometimes, it is intimacy that is missing, and this can lead to a feeling of disconnection that makes it more difficult to desire and enjoy sex. You ask yourself, "Why should I? He doesn't care about me until he wants something from me." The opposite can also be true. Sometimes, we may only desire intimacy and not sex. We want the closeness and connection but not necessarily the mechanics of it all. It is okay if you desire this at times; however, if this is the only way you want to connect with your partner, there may be some issues that need to be addressed.

The security of a committed relationship can make sex an incredibly freeing experience because you know your partner is in it for the long haul and is not going anywhere. Your partner knows you and what you like and that special spot that always gets you going. However, familiarity can be a two-edged sword if complacency sets in, and there is no excitement and variety. Good sex requires some novelty even if it's just switching up the time of day you do the deed.

Being receptive is also important for having good sex. Women who struggle with low or no sex drive are less likely to be able to distinguish when they are aroused and when they are not. This presents a problem for receptivity if you are not even aware of when you do want sex. Even if you are not having any problems with low sex drive, your brain can sometimes make being receptive difficult. Have you ever been approached by your partner for sex only to remember how they snapped at you earlier in the day, and your desire came to a screeching halt? Our logic and reasoning can enhance or dampen our willingness to engage in sexual activity.

Commonly, when we think about sex, we envision it occurring with a partner. However, you can cultivate intimacy and enjoy sex by yourself. Developing a close and personal relationship with yourself is so important to your overall health and well-being. Woman, know thyself! To know you is to love you...seriously! Engaging in activities that promote self-exploration and personal development are the keys to learning more about who you are. Consider dating yourself. Spending quality time alone can uncover many things that you didn't know about yourself. And, side note, you may find that you enjoy taking yourself out to dinner and a movie. You may find that you enjoy your own company. Loving you is an important piece to establish before getting into a relationship; otherwise, you run the risk of becoming codependent.

As I said before, sex can be enjoyed as a solo sport. Now, don't get me wrong when I say that partnered sex is good, but it can be helpful to engage in self-play or masturbation in order to discover the activities, thoughts, and sensations that turn you on. You get to figure out what you like and what gives you pleasure. You also have the opportunity to try different things without having to worry about your partner agreeing to do it. There is a certain freedom that comes with self-play. You can just allow your reactions to flow uncensored because you are not worried about how you look or sound to someone else.

Notes

Notes

Notes

Notes

_____

_____

_____

_____

_____

_____

_____

_____

_____

_____

_____

_____

_____

_____

_____

_____

_____

_____

_____

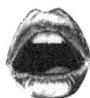

CHAPTER 3

WHEN TO GET HELP

Your level of sexual desire is not always constant. It changes. A lot. It all depends on what is happening in your life. Many women will come in asking for hormone testing when this happens, believing that she is going into menopause when her desire for sex starts to dip. She is convinced her estrogen and testosterone are low. Usually, this information is obtained from a well-meaning friend or older family member. Now, it is good to have someone you can go to for information and advice about these issues. However, it is important that the source is reputable and is knowledgeable. Generally speaking, there is so much misinformation out there about women's reproductive health, menstrual periods, hormones, menopause, and sex specifically. Often when women come in for problems dealing with sex and desire, it is found to be a symptom of some underlying issue. It tends to show up during times of life transitions like getting married, pregnancy and having a baby, getting divorced, and menopause.

Problems with sex and desire can be associated with many other causes. Fatigue is the number one reason most women give as to why they don't want to have sex. Our schedules are so jam-packed with activities during the day and often late into the night. We are taking care of our kids while simultaneously caring for aging parents or stressed about how we are going to pay for college and long-term care. We are not sleeping well due to the stress, and because we have our cell phones and computers in our faces stimulating us right up until we fall asleep, it is even worse. And there is this underlying perception that if you take a break, you are a failure.

Certain medical conditions may also predispose you to having problems with sex and desire. The list includes a broad spectrum of diseases including hypertension, diabetes, urinary incontinence, neurological diseases like multiple sclerosis (MS), premature ovarian failure, menopause, cancers (especially breast or gynecologic cancers), depression, and anxiety. You are also more likely to have issues with sex if you have had any significant trauma like sexual molestation, abuse or rape, genital mutilation, been in a relationship characterized by domestic violence, or have problems with substance abuse. Relationship discord and stress, whether it is emotional or environmental, can make it more difficult to desire sex or to have an orgasm. Some women also have issues with sex due to their cultural or religious teachings. Even certain medications can cause problems with sex and desire. Medications to treat high blood pressure, mood disorders like depression and anxiety, and even antihistamines can all be implicated in women's struggles with sex and desire. Even with that long list of potential reasons, it is not unusual for sexual dysfunction to show up at times when everything seems to be going great, your relationship is good, you're not stressed, and no particular cause can be found.

With so many potential physical, emotional, mental, and spiritual causes of sexual dysfunction in women, where would you start to try and unravel the issue and get help if you need it? Your doctor? Sure. Your primary care doctor or your gynecologist? Or maybe you need a therapist? Well, I'll tell you that most doctors are not well-versed in diagnosing and treating problems in women. The most training that I got while in medical school was how to take a sexual history and how to screen for sexually transmitted infections (STIs). Add to that the fact that a significant number of doctors do not feel comfortable asking their patients about their sex life and if they are happy with it. The taboo is real! But on the other side, many women do not feel comfortable with sharing their questions and concerns with their doctor. As a physician with education in this area, I make it a point to ask about sexual problems during the normal course of a well-woman visit. But not all doctors will pursue any additional training in this area, and as such, are not comfortable with inquiring about sexual health beyond asking about sexual history and STIs because they are afraid of opening Pandora's box. They don't know what to do with what comes out. And you, as the patient, may feel embarrassed to bring the subject up during the course of your exam.

But, do me a favor? If you decide to ask your doctor a question about your sexual concerns, PLEASE, do not wait until your visit is over and the doctor has their hand on the doorknob, to mention it. I know that it may take that long to gather your courage to ask. The problem with this strategy is the answer you need is rarely a quick line or two of instructions. We need time and space to fully evaluate the characteristics of the issue and relay the treatment plan to you. You wouldn't wait until the end of your visit to tell your doctor that you are having chest pain, so don't do it for sexual concerns either. Okay, I'm getting down off of my soapbox.

So, it still begs the question of who can you see for help with low sex drive or sexual dysfunction in women? Historically, this has been the territory of therapists-conventional therapists as well as sex therapists, or a sexologist. There has recently been an increase in the life coaching industry, and some coaches concentrate on helping with relationship and sex issues. There have also been inroads made in traditional medicine with more physicians who are interested in learning more about and treating women's problems with sex and desire. If you are able to see a physician with this special skill set, you would have the added benefit of being able to rule out a physical cause for your sexual concerns as well as creating a treatment plan to address it.

Because there are several options for evaluation, how do you decide who to see? Often, you will need to see at least a physician to rule out and/or address any physical cause for the problem. And then you can decide if you feel that you need more support in this area with a therapist or a life coach.

Notes

Notes

_____

_____

_____

_____

_____

_____

_____

_____

_____

_____

_____

_____

_____

_____

_____

_____

_____

_____

_____

Notes

Notes

_____

_____

_____

_____

_____

_____

_____

_____

_____

_____

_____

_____

_____

_____

_____

_____

_____

_____

_____

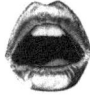

CHAPTER 4

CHANGING YOUR MINDSET

The brain is your biggest sex organ, so it makes sense that we would start here discussing how to transform your sex life. Sex is so important that it is hardwired into the brain. We know that one reason is that sex is necessary for the propagation of our species, for our continued existence on this planet. With such a critical role, it is considered a basic physiological need.

Abraham Maslow, the American psychologist who developed the Theory of Human Motivation, determined that human achievement is predicated on fulfilling innate human needs. And according to Maslow's hierarchy of needs, sex shows up on several levels. Sex is a basic need and is at the foundation or bottom of the pyramid along with food, water, and sleep. Sex is controlled and regulated by one of the oldest parts of the brain, the same place where many of our drives and desires to obtain food and water- to breathe even, are regulated.

Maslow's theory said that in order to move up to the higher levels of achievement, the needs of the lower levels had to be sufficiently met.

So, we have the basic needs of food, water, sleep, and sex on level 1.

Moving up the pyramid of Maslow's hierarchy, sex shows up again under sense of safety - as a security of body. In order for a woman to have sex, she has to feel comfortable, safe, and secure. Certain portions of her brain related to fear have to be turned down or off for her to have and enjoy sex and orgasm.

Sexual intimacy satisfies our need for love and belonging. That's on level 3.

Self-esteem and confidence are also affected and influenced by sex, and that's level 4.

Your own flair, finesse, and style are influenced by your comfort level with sex.

The top of the pyramid is self-actualization, and sex shows up there in our creativity and problem-solving skills. Your power, wit, and ingenuity are all interwoven with sex.

So, now you know that your brain is hardwired for sex! It is your biggest sex organ. But it can work against you.

The oldest parts of the brain, what would be called the reptilian brain, controls basic drives and desires, and like I've told you, sex is one of those. It's a reflex!

However, the newer parts of the brain, the limbic brain and neocortex, the parts that have to do with emotion, logic, and reasoning can modulate your response to your basic drives. Something as simple as being able to wait for a bathroom break to relieve yourself during a meeting, instead of going as soon as you feel the urge is one example of how this process works.

Another example would be feeling turned on when you see your partner doing the dishes, and having an overwhelming sense of love and desire for sex because you see that he cares enough to help you with the household chores. Whatever emotions are triggered by what is happening around you influences your motivation to act on it - and that can mean stuffing the desire or being open to moving forward and taking action to satisfy that desire.

Knowing that the brain plays such a large part in sexual desire and arousal, what does the female sexual response cycle look like? In contrast to men, it has a circular orientation as opposed to a linear orientation. For men, it goes in a straight line from desire to arousal to orgasm to plateau. For women, it is a more complex dance, and there are several paths to desire and orgasm and many ways to achieve spontaneous sexual desire. Things like emotional intimacy and emotional, mental, and physical satisfaction play a part in a woman's ability to achieve sexual desire. However, she can start from a place of sexual neutrality and still get there.

Another challenge faced by women is identifying when their sex drive has shown up and when she is aroused. Women can become indifferent to sex as it slips further and further down the priority list. As you go about your day, you may miss cues from your body that you are receptive to sex or that you are aroused. Several studies were done to see if women who identify as having low sex drive could tell when they were aroused using objective measurements (increased heart rate, increased breathing, vaginal lubrication, and increased vaginal blood flow), and they found that these women did not recognize the signs of arousal even though their bodies were experiencing them. How awful! You can forget what it feels like to be aroused!

It is also possible to confuse the signals you are getting. Like we discussed earlier, sex is tied into areas of the brain responsible for drives, desires, and satisfaction. And the same places that are activated when you have, say a piece of chocolate, is the same place that is activated when you think about and have sex. So, sometimes, we can confuse our desire for sex as a desire for feel-good foods like chocolate, ice cream, cakes, or pies. It can also be confused with things that give you an endorphin rush, those feel-good hormones like dopamine. So, you may be feeling that "itch" but substituting, successfully substituting, other things that satisfy in a similar way.

At one point in my married life when both my husband and I were working hard to grow our businesses and were barely seeing each other, I began to have a strange craving. I am not a fan of chocolate, but I began craving chocolate cake. The first time I didn't think anything about it, but it kept happening. After a bit, I began to question what was underneath the craving. What came to me was that I was actually desiring sex, but the craving for chocolate cake was how it manifested.

———

We already talked about novelty as a component of good sex. When you were younger or at the beginning of your relationship, sex was new, exciting, and fun, but after a while, especially with the same partner, it became ho-hum and boring. So why have it? Why do it? It takes so much effort to get "in the mood" and for what?

Changing the outside or environmental factors like timing or location can inject novelty. But you can also create change by establishing new neural pathways in your brain. When we think about the creation of new neural pathways, we think that it is limited to young babies and children. However, your brain is like a computer or smartphone. Just like we update the operating system for our electronics, we can update the operating system for our brains, including for sex. You can add more of what you want, and take out the things that you don't want. One way to create fertile ground for a new neural pathway is meditation. There is a lot of noise in our daily lives, so taking time to quiet our minds can allow us to listen to our inner voice. It can be uncomfortable to be quiet with yourself at first. It feels uncomfortable to sit and do what seems like nothing. Your inner mean girl will have lots to say in that empty space. Your true inner voice may be harder to hear, although she will likely have a lot to say about what is happening with your sex drive. By allowing for quiet, you are giving her permission to speak to you. You are telling her that you are open and listening to what she has to say.

Once you are meditating, you can more easily access your subconscious mind for change and begin to update your operating system. Journaling is a great way to explore what is currently running in your brain's operating system. The first step to change is awareness. You have to know what is already there before you can alter it. The key to journaling is 1) doing it consistently, and 2) getting out all of the top-of-mind things first, like the stuff you need to put on your to-do list. Next, you want to begin journaling around specific prompts or questions. Some examples include:

- What five things gave you pleasure today?
- In what ways are you loving and nurturing yourself?
- What lights you up? What makes you excited?
- Do you agree or disagree with this statement: *I have permission to feel pleasure?*
- What do you like about sex?
- What do you hate about sex?

Don't forget to meditate for a few minutes before you begin the journaling session to access your subconscious mind. Try not to edit what you are writing. Just let the thoughts and feelings flow.

How easy was it for you to write out five things that gave you pleasure every day? Did your answers to the other prompts surprise you?

―――――

Do you know your natural sex cycle – how often you desire sex? Are you so used to saying no that your sex cycle is set to never? Your body has a rhythm that is unique for you and is dependent on many factors that can throw off your rhythm or distract you from recognizing your body's signals. Sex is a vital part of how you show up in the world. Knowing your rhythm allows you to honor it. Notice when your mind wanders to sexy thoughts or even when you are aware of certain sensations like your blouse gliding across your skin. This is the beginning of recognizing your body's signals for sex. You also want to be aware of what may be blocking you from acknowledging your sensual thoughts and sensations. By attuning to both, you are working toward creating balance in your life around sex. You are better able to know when you want to have sex and when you are just saying no out of habit.

Notes

Notes

Notes

Notes

CHAPTER 5

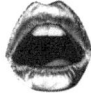

BRING THE PLEASURE

Now that you have prepared your mind to create new neural pathways, it is time to create new habits around sex and pleasure. The key to doing this is by creating experiences. Remember Dorothy and the Technicolor lesson. Creating experiences is what takes you from a black and white existence, just following the routine, with no excitement or anticipation for what is coming next. We've got to get you out of the rut. Sir Isaac Newton's first law of motion states that if an object is at rest it will stay at rest unless an external force acts on it. Let this be your external force to get you moving again.

We talked about the importance of being receptive to pleasure, but that can be more of a passive activity. I want you to be more active and invite pleasure into your life. How do you do that? First, by making a decision that you will have a pleasurable life. And then paying attention to the things that show up and bring you pleasure. Now, this doesn't have to be sexual at all. It could be basking in the feel of the hot water on your skin as you shower. It could be enjoying a good belly laugh with a coworker. It could be experiencing a moving piece of artwork. Pleasure is not restricted to the bedroom, nor should it be. You can get curious and begin to notice what brings you pleasure.

Even when you are doing routine things, you can look for the pleasure in them. Sometimes this can be a bit challenging but the rewards are that it gives you a more positive outlook on life and makes you feel good. "Will this bring me pleasure?" is a great question to ask yourself throughout the day. If the answer is yes, do it full out. If the answer is no, think about a simple way to bring pleasure to the activity. A drive to the grocery store can be livened up with a little karaoke, James Corden style.

Once you get the hang of inviting pleasure into your life, the next step is to begin to look for signs of sexual desire and arousal. Remember, I told you that the less you pay attention to your sexual desire and arousal, the less it will show up. Developing a practice of noticing signs of desire and arousal can be as simple as appreciating the appearance of a handsome man, noticing when you are having any thoughts of a sexual nature (no matter how fleeting), or noting any genital tingling or lubrication. Then acknowledge and celebrate these wins. The more you notice and acknowledge these occurrences and bring positive energy around them, the more you are reprogramming your mind to keep showing them to you.

Now, the next step is creating pleasurable sexual experiences. When something is pleasurable, we usually want to do it again and again. But even if the sex is good, sometimes it can be difficult to get into a place of being open to it. Amping up the whole experience can be a way to get you more engaged and excited for sex. The movies do have one part right, it is important to set the mood. And this doesn't always have to mean low lights or candles and soft music. Your idea of a fun time may include a strobe light or disco ball, and if that's the case, go for it! I think the single most important rule is to make sure you engage the five senses. The more of these that are stimulated, the better the chance of you having and remembering this pleasurable experience. So pick a theme, then decorate your space. You can use costumes. You can have sexy snacks and play up the texture and temperature differences. This can also be done with fabrics and linens. Diffuse essential oils with erotic fragrances. Use music or ambient sounds to transport you to a different place. Keep thinking, *"Yes that would be good, and what else is possible to make this fun, exciting, or more pleasurable?"*

My final directive is: have more sex! Getting creative and having a more positive experience with sex will create the desire for more of it. Having more sex can also provide you with more opportunities to evaluate what is happening throughout the encounters. You can see what patterns there are around how your partner approaches you for sex, how you approach your partner for sex, how the actual episode plays out, and what happens during the afterglow period. I want you to use it as an opportunity to be a detective and identify what you like or don't like about each aspect. DO NOT analyze all three parts during the same sexual encounter; just pick one. It is too distracting to monitor the whole thing, and you are likely not to enjoy anything at all if you are evaluating everything. One final note, if you ARE NOT interested in sex, please do not force yourself to have sex. There will be more on this in Chapter 10, but if you are not open to sex or turned on, you can be making the situation worse instead of better by "taking one for the team."

Notes

Notes

Notes

Notes

CHAPTER 6

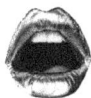

DO YOU KNOW
YOUR ANATOMY?

Any good book on sex should have a section on anatomy. The reason is that the vulva and vagina are a mystery to many women. And if you don't know what is down there, how can you hope to maximize your pleasure? It is important to remember that this is just a diagram. Every woman is unique and may have slightly different anatomy.

So, how can you use your anatomy to your advantage for enjoying sex and having orgasms? The first thing to do is to get familiar with your own anatomy. Take a look at your body. Your whole body. Yes, there are certain spots that have a larger concentration of nerve endings that can be stimulated to give pleasure, but your whole body is involved in sexual desire and pleasure and should be included in this exploration. A full-length mirror works best for looking at your entire body at one time, but a handheld mirror is a better choice when you begin a more intimate exploration of your genital area. See if you can identify some of the structures pictured in the diagram on yourself.

Female external reproductive organs

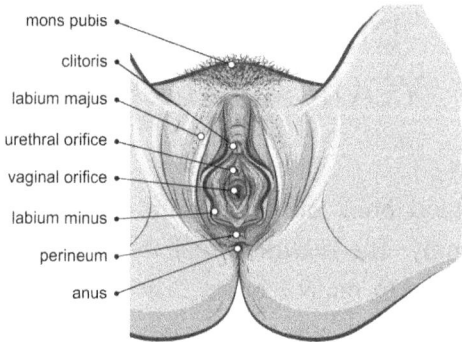

mons pubis
clitoris
labium majus
urethral orifice
vaginal orifice
labium minus
perineum
anus

Female Reproductive System

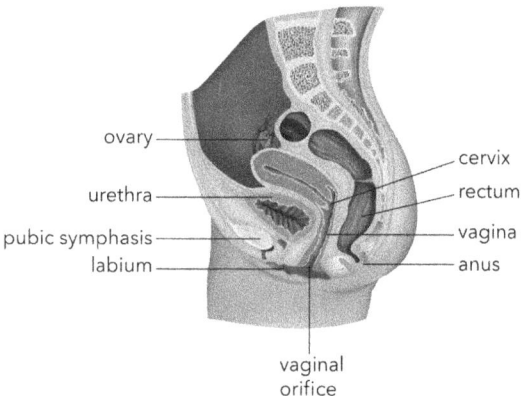

ovary
urethra
pubic symphasis
labium

cervix
rectum
vagina
anus

vaginal orifice

Once you feel like you have sufficiently studied where things are and what they look like, it is time to move on to touching these areas. Get curious and explore the sensations of touching areas that you were able to name, maybe for the first time. Try and see if you can find your G-spot. There is some debate about whether or not the G-spot really exists. And if you have been unsuccessful in being able to find it and stimulate it, you, too, may believe that it is an elusive unicorn. For those of us who do believe that it exists, it is typically described as being located on the "front wall" of the vagina about an inch inside of the opening. Keep in mind that the texture of the vaginal tissues in this area feels different from the surrounding vagina and may give you a clue that you've found it. Eureka!

Touch your clitoris. That little nubbin of tissue is not the entirety of the clitoris; it is just the most visible part. The clitoris occupies a much larger area than most people know and has legs! Try stroking the outer labia. This can produce sensations that are just as pleasurable as if you were stroking the clitoris, but generally, they are less intense. Touch the perineum. Stimulating this area can also produce sensations of pleasure. There are so many places on your body that can be a source of pleasure if you take the time to get to know them.

Here comes the brain again. Have you ever found yourself reflecting back on a prior pleasurable sexual encounter and getting all hot and bothered like it was happening right then? Reflecting back on past experiences and even using fantasy is another way to explore the largest pleasure point in your body, your brain. Your brain doesn't know the difference between what is really happening and what you are seeing with your mind's eye. The same neurons fire, the same feel-good chemicals are released, and you can even orgasm just from the mental stimulation. Fantasizing and visualizing can also be powerful tools to initially explore some of the more taboo sexual adventures that you are thinking about trying. You may be surprised at what you find you like and what turns you on, and the fantasy realm allows you to try something out before you attempt it in real life. If you have never done this, set aside some time and try it. Let your mind flow where it wants and allow the sensations to course through your body. If you feel comfortable, and you have a favorite fantasy, you can ask your partner to help you recreate it.

Now that you know the anatomy, and have had some exploration time, can we talk about orgasms? How many different types of orgasms do you think there are? Two? Four? There are at least 10 different types of orgasms available through stimulation of various places on your body. You are probably familiar with those attributed to the clitoris. Many women are only able to orgasm through clitoral stimulation. But what about the other spots? It is likely that neither the women or their partners know about them or how to stimulate them.

And what is an orgasm anyway? If that scene in "When Harry Met Sally" comes to mind, you are not alone. Even though Sally was faking, this is how most people envision an orgasm to be. The technical definition of an orgasm is the sudden release of built-up sexual excitement, resulting in rhythmic muscle contractions in the pelvic region that is characterized by sexual pleasure. Although we have a succinct definition for what an orgasm is, it is important to note that orgasms are not all alike nor are they one-size-fits-all. They can be experienced differently by different women and also have different manifestations in the same woman. You may have an explosive, earth-shattering experience that leaves you breathless and invigorated one time. The next time it may be an experience with less fireworks but with a warmth that flows over your body leaving you feeling complete and serene. Another time, you may feel like you've had a spiritual experience, like you have connected with the divine and have gained a deeper knowledge of the universe. Physiologically, we know what an orgasm is, but it is so much more than its physical manifestation.

Notes

Notes

Notes

Notes

_____

_____

_____

_____

_____

_____

_____

_____

_____

_____

_____

_____

_____

_____

_____

_____

_____

_____

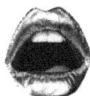

CHAPTER 7

MORE PLEASURE PLEASE

Now that you are having sex, I think it is only right that we talk about ways to heighten and extend your pleasure from sex. One of the ways to do this is by strengthening the muscles of your pelvic floor. Why does this help? It allows you to have more control. The pleasure from intercourse generally relies on applied friction. During intercourse, you can voluntarily contract your pelvic floor muscles, causing increased friction, and thereby increase pleasure. By that same token, you can increase the intensity and sometimes the duration of an orgasm by strengthening the muscles of the pelvic floor. These same muscles contract during orgasm and remember that an orgasm is the rhythmic contraction of the muscles in the pelvic region that is characterized by sexual pleasure. If the muscles are stronger, they can contract with more intensity and produce more intense pleasure.

So, how do you strengthen these muscles? You can do pelvic floor exercises (Kegel exercises) to help improve their strength. The exercises involve contracting the muscles and holding them in a contracted state for a few seconds, followed by a short rest. The more of these that you do, the better the control and strength you will have. You can identify which muscles you should be contracting by paying attention to what muscles you use to stop the flow of urine when you go to the bathroom. If you are clenching your butt muscles or tensing your abdominal muscles, you are not doing it correctly. There are now pelvic floor exercisers available to help you with doing these exercises. Some of them are doubly helpful because they use vibration to give you feedback on when to squeeze and how hard to squeeze, but the vibrations can also stimulate sexual arousal.

Although the key to pleasure from intercourse relies on applied friction, using a lubricant can add to your pleasure as well. Dry skin rubbing on dry skin is horrible. Think fingernails on chalkboard horrible. Lubricants can ease the way if you are not making enough lubrication on your own, but be careful not to use too much, otherwise, all the friction is gone, and you may not feel anything. I recommend using a water-based or silicone-based product, as they are less likely to cause an imbalance inside of the vagina or cause infection. There are specialty lubricants that have a warming or cooling feature. These can increase the sensitivity of the genital tissues, increasing your chances of orgasming. However, do not use too much, as the same ingredients that help in a small amount can actually hurt you and make your genitals very uncomfortable in larger amounts.

There are also creams and gels that can help get you in the mood and heighten pleasure through different means. Gels like Zestra and scream cream or passion cream helps to increase blood flow to the genital area. This increase in blood flow not only allows for more friction because the genital tissues are fuller, but they can also cause an increase in your natural production of lubrication. The increased blood flow also translates into increased sensitivity of the tissues to stimulation, making orgasms easier to attain.

Prolonging orgasm is also a thing. The practice is called *edging*. It is achieved through sexual stimulation to the point right before you orgasm, and then the stimulation is stopped and you breathe deeply until you feel like you can receive more sexual stimulation. And you do it again and again, building the height of pleasure until you are ready to experience the climax. This practice involves a great deal of control because you have to be able to get so close to the orgasm without going too far, either inadvertently or intentionally because it feels so good.

The use of adult toys can also add to your heightened pleasure. There are so many different types available you would be hard-pressed not to find something you like. There are vibrating ones, some specifically designed to stimulate the clitoris and the G-spot. There are ones that don't vibrate but mimic a penis to be used for penetration. There are ones that can be used with a partner during sex as well. If you want to explore anal stimulation, there are other accessories that are helpful for that. Whichever type you choose, make sure to look for a reputable brand that uses medical-grade silicone. It is important that the parts meant to touch or enter the sensitive genital area are "cast" or created in a single piece. This is because if it is cast in more than one piece and then assembled, there can be unfinished edges that can cut you. Also, the seam where the parts come together can be a source of infection, as it can be difficult to clean it properly. Always follow the instructions provided with the toy for the proper use and care, cleaning, and storage of it, so that it can stand the test of time.

Let's talk about other supplements that can enhance your sexual experience. Cannabidiol may have some benefit for some women in the bedroom. The research shows conflicting data regarding the effect of cannabinoids, of which cannabidiol (CBD) is one, on sexual desire and pleasure. We do know that the relaxing, anti-anxiety properties of this substance can facilitate a woman being more receptive to sexual activity. The analgesic effects can also help women who experience pain with sexual activity. CBD can be consumed in a number of ways, which affects how quickly you can feel the effects as well as the potential side effects. Lubricants containing CBD can be absorbed through the skin and mucosal surface of the vagina fairly easily. Use should be guided by the instructions on the packaging, and CBD lube can be applied at any time during the sexual act. Caution should be observed when using CBD lube with sex toys, as with other lubes, because it can degrade the toy material. Another concern is that although CBD lube is applied locally to the genitals, it can have some systemic absorption. Anyone taking certain medications for depression or mood changes, seizures/epilepsy, blood thinners, or any medications that call for them to avoid consuming grapefruit, should avoid CBD lube. There can be an increase in the blood levels of these medications leading to dangerous side effects.

Here's another unicorn for you: multiple orgasms. There are two ways to think about having multiple orgasms. The first is as a linear or sequential fashion. This just means that one orgasm follows another (and another and another if you're lucky). For women, there is very little refractory period or downtime between having one orgasm and being able to enjoy another, so this makes intuitive sense. The second is orgasms occurring concurrently. This means that you have stimulation of multiple areas of the body that create intense feelings of pleasure in these multiple areas, with you climaxing altogether at one time. I'm not sure if this second one actually should be categorized as a blended orgasm, but I would still go for it.

Notes

Notes

Notes

Notes

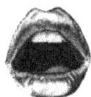

CHAPTER 8

SEX IS SELF-CARE

All bodies are capable of good sex and orgasm no matter their size, shape, or weight! Let me say that again! All bodies are capable of good sex and orgasm no matter their size, shape, or weight. Even as we are seeing more realistic representations of women's bodies in media and print, there is still a pervasive image of beauty being represented by a woman who is thin, with small breasts and minimal hips/butts. But this is not what the average woman looks like. She has some curves, and she is not a stick figure. But regardless of your body shape, everyone has the same systems within their bodies. We are all hardwired to be able to have pleasure and enjoy sex.

Do you love your body? Most women would say no, or they start to name off all the parts of their body that they don't like when asked that question. Even when someone compliments a woman, do you notice how she will deflect it instead of accepting it? We are painfully aware of our flaws and don't want anyone to give us credit when we feel like it is not due. Your inner mean girl will ridicule you about the weight you need to lose, the way that your skin hangs on your arms, even the shape of your eyebrows. Why? Because she/we are comparing ourselves to other women, and we will always find ourselves lacking. Guess what? There is no competition! You are fearfully and wonderfully made and uniquely you! There is no one like you, so there is no one with whom you can effectively compare yourself.

What would it look like for you to love your body? What would you say to yourself in the mirror? In our heads, we all have an inner dialogue running all the time. And that inner dialogue is generally pessimistic and driven by the ego that is trying to protect us from some perceived threat to our sense of self and safety. In that context, it makes sense why women will try to compare themselves to other women and take steps to fit in. We need to stay in the group. It is hardwired in our DNA because evolutionarily being in a community or in a group ensured your safety and survival. Even though we are out of the Stone Ages, community is still important to our sense of well-being and how we identify ourselves. I believe that it is possible to be a part of a group and manage your inner dialogue to work in your favor. What would it look like if you had a more positive and inspiring inner dialogue running through your head? How would that change how you show up in the world?

The first step to change is awareness. I want you to become aware of the inner thoughts going through your mind during the day. If you are doing an activity and you make a mistake, what do you hear about yourself in your mind? Is it something like, "you're stupid" or "that was a dumb mistake?" If you hear things like this, I want you to counteract it with truth. Say, "I am not stupid and this was a simple mistake," and then move on. Things happen, and they are generally neutral, but we like to assign meaning to them. By reframing the meaning, you take away the negative charge and begin to make way for at least neutrality if not positivity of it.

The next level would be to start adding more positive thoughts to your inner dialogue. How do you do that? Surround yourself with positivity. What you put in is what comes out. Positive people, inspirational quotes, listening to podcasts, and reading books that are uplifting, are all great strategies for increasing the positivity factor.

Another way to add positivity to your life is to begin taking good care of yourself. We all know that we should treat our bodies right, but we don't generally do it. We understand that taking care of ourselves is a good idea, yadda yadda yadda, but it never quite makes the cut. So really, why should we do it? Strictly from a physiological standpoint, our bodies are made to operate within a small range of acceptable conditions and staying within these ranges helps our bodies to function optimally. Our bodies are made up of about 70 percent water (and our brains are even more water dominant). So, when we ingest enough water, we are helping our bodies to function optimally.

The same goes for sleep. Sleep deprivation not only kills your desire for but your enjoyment of sex as well. If sex does happen, you may be thinking to yourself, *"I can't wait till this is over, so I can go to sleep."* You are cheating yourself out of the wonderful experience that great sex can be. When you are well-rested, you are able to be present in the moment, attuned to the wonderful sensations that come from touching and being touched. Your mind is freed up to be more creative, and you are free to be adventurous because you aren't limited by physical fatigue. When your body does not regenerate properly, something has to give.

Other forms of taking care of your body are moving your body and eating good foods that don't make you feel sluggish and bloated. Often, as we get older, we do not move as much as we used to as children. We have certain activities that we do, and our routines do not change. It is important to change things up and move your body in different ways. Specifically, activities that involve moving the pelvis can help. Movements like those done in belly dancing bring awareness to how you are moving your hips and pelvis. We need to engage these muscles, so they are not stiff and can move fluidly. This will help when you are trying new positions in the bedroom. The movement also helps to increase blood flow to the tissues in the pelvis, including the genitals. And, the added benefit if you pick a "sexy" type of dance to do, you are engaging all of your senses and increasing the likelihood of at least feeling sexy even if you're not having or pursuing sexual activity. It also will give you a better sense of how your body relates to the space that it is in.

For me, I like dance classes because they are fun, it doesn't feel like a structured exercise regimen, and I am moving parts of my body that I don't usually engage in a normal day. You may be surprised at what your body can do. It has not forgotten how to move, and it can be encouraged to move out of your comfort zones. Trying something new can increase your confidence and feelings of self-esteem too. If you are not into dance, try yoga or sign up to play a team sport. The point is to get moving in a way that is different from the norm.

Having sex is a great way to treat your body well. Yes, sex is a form of self-care. Self-care is defined as any activity that refuels or replenishes you and doesn't drain you. It is "anything that we do deliberately in order to take care of our mental, emotional, and physical health . . . Good self-care is key to improved mood and reduced anxiety. It's also key to a good relationship with oneself and others" (R. Michael, MA, "What Self-Care Is—and

What It Isn't," Psych Central Online, July 8, 2018, https://psychcentral.com/blog/what-self-care-is-and-what-it-isnt-2/).

Sex definitely falls under this definition. It is known to improve mood, decrease stress and anxiety, decrease pain, increase your creativity and problem-solving skills, and increase your sense of connection, and improve relationships when it is practiced regularly. My prescription for you is to begin to think of having sex as taking good care of yourself and to engage in it regularly. A survey conducted on sexual activity in couples found that the happiest couples were the ones who were having sex at least once a week. You can consider making that your goal to start with.

Notes

Notes

Notes

Notes

CHAPTER 9

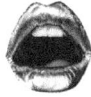

CONFIDENTLY SEXY

Before we begin discussing being sexy and confident, I think it is important to define what it is and what it is not. For me, being sexy simply means being confident in your own skin. It is knowing that you are awesome just as you are but you are also doing the work to grow because you know that you have greater potential. Being sexy is not about being overly sexual or overly aggressive. It is not doing things to get the attention of the opposite sex. And although it does not have a direct role in attracting potential partners, if you are confident and sexy, you are more likely to be attractive to potential partners.

Being confident and sexy includes having a sense of being able to handle any challenge that may come your way. It is so easy to forget how much we have overcome already, and we start to doubt our ability to handle life. But think back on a time when you had a challenge. How did you overcome it? Whatever happened, you handled it, and you are here to tell the tale of it. You survived it. Those are the things that confidence is made of. Another way to increase your confidence is to engage in new experiences and activities or to pursue a new hobby, talent, or dream. Once you do these things, you will gain a sense of your own capabilities and begin to see what else is possible for you when you get out of your comfort zone.

You can be confident and sexy in the bedroom. Again, it doesn't have to mean that you are overly aggressive or overly sexualized (unless you want to be). There are many reasons that women do not show up confident and sexy in the bedroom. One reason is that a woman may not "own" the fact that sex is supposed to be a pleasurable experience for her as well as her partner. She may feel like being confident and sexy means she has to be in the driver's seat, directing what is happening, which can be intimidating. It may represent a departure from the "good girl" image that we've grown up with, implying that there are some things that a "good girl" doesn't do. She may be afraid that she won't be able to control the episode, and will be forced to continue on in an activity even if she gets uncomfortable and wants to stop.

Just as you can build confidence, there are certain things that can break it down. One thing that can erode your confidence is when you either do not have boundaries or you don't enforce those boundaries. Now, I know what you may be thinking. You just said to be open to trying new things and having new experiences. But now you want to talk about boundaries and non-negotiables? Yes. This is not an *either/or* conversation. This is a *yes/and* conversation. When you don't have or enforce your boundaries and non-negotiables, it usually means that you are not sure of who you are and what you stand for, or you don't want to disappoint or hurt another person. You are more likely to go along with what someone else wants or suggests if you don't already know what you want and need. With respect to sex, this is especially important. You have to be aware of what you want and don't want. This includes something as basic as consent to engage in sex and extends to being able to navigate requests you make of your partner and those requests made of you by your partner. So yes, be open to trying new things and having new experiences but only to the extent and degree that you feel comfortable and not used or degraded.

Notes

Notes

Notes

Notes

_____
_____
_____
_____
_____
_____
_____
_____
_____
_____
_____
_____
_____
_____
_____
_____
_____
_____
_____

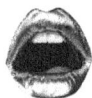

CHAPTER 10

WHAT ABOUT YOUR PARTNER?

So, now that you have all of this information, how do you interact with your partner and bring them along for the journey? I would suggest sitting down with them and having a discussion about what is happening with you. You can express your experience with sex and intimacy and talk about how it makes you feel when you don't desire sex with your partner. Being open and honest is a good way to start the conversation. Let them know that the reason you are taking action is because you care about them and the state of the relationship including the sexual aspect of it. Let them know you want to see things improve and are willing to do your part to make that happen. Then ask if they are willing to help you along the journey. Most likely, they will say yes. (If they say no, that's a whole other conversation that needs to happen.) It is then important for you to give some guidance on how they can support you. One area they can support you is in demonstrating patience with you and the process. Change does not happen overnight. You didn't get here in five minutes, and it will take longer than five minutes to reprogram your thoughts and behaviors. Another important piece will be a willingness to engage in physical touch and intimacy-generating activities for the sake of touch and not as a means to an end to get sex. Thirdly, ask your partner if he is willing to hear feedback about how he can tweak his approach, performance, or post-sex game. Reassure him it will not be delivered in a harsh way nor is it meant to place blame on him.

A common area of contention in partnered sex has to do with initiation and refusal. This can be challenging because as women we typically see ourselves as being on the receiving end of sexual advances. We have to determine if we are open to sexual activity or not. Listen to your intuition where this is concerned. I like to use the analogy of a traffic light to demonstrate how to gauge where you are on the sexual response curve. Sometimes you know that you are just not in the mood, and so in those instances, you would refuse the advance. This would be a red light. However, a lot of times, women are in a sex-neutral state. This means that they are not overtly open to sexual arousal but not overtly closed to it either. This would be a yellow light. And those times when you have an enthusiastic yes to sexual arousal would be a green light. Once you have identified where you are, you can respond to the initiation attempt. But wherever you find yourself, honor that.

When you are a yellow light or sex-neutral, things can go either way - you can speed up to get to the green light, or you can slow down to the red light. To move from yellow to green, you will likely need a little time and more stimulation. When I say a little time, I mean like 15 minutes, not 15 years. You will use that time to move into a sex-yes state. Sometimes, it's as simple as going to take a quick shower and changing your clothes to something more comfortable. Other times, you may need to go and listen to some sensual music and move your hips or dance to get things moving in the right direction. You could also read or listen to an erotic story or engage in some solo sex play before joining your partner. Your partner can also be a part of this process. If you need some extra physical touch from your partner, let them know. A little hand-holding or some passionate kissing can turn the tide and make things hot and heavy.

Another challenge around initiating is that often one partner is always the one to initiate sex, and they dream of their partner initiating sex sometimes. It makes them feel like you don't desire them if you are not asking for or initiating sex even if you are having sex with them when they do initiate a sexual advance. So, sometimes, you will have to initiate sex. That can be as simple as a wink at the dinner table. It can be as elaborate as a treasure hunt around the house until your partner finds you ready and waiting to have some fun.

Now that we've talked about initiation, let's talk about refusal. In the context of a love relationship, you still have the right to have and enforce your boundaries around when you want to have sex and when you don't. But it does not stop there. You have the right to have and enforce boundaries around the type of sexual activity that you will engage in. The most important thing is communication. You have to communicate to your partner what you are and are not willing to do. You can decide to try something new but know that you are not obligated to continue with that something new just because your partner wants you to do it. Sex is a two-way street, and it is intended for both parties to receive pleasure from it. If you are doing something that you do not want to do, that is not pleasurable, you can and should stop.

Speaking of refusal, what happens when a couple has a mismatch of sexual desire? There can be a breakdown in the relationship sometimes to the point of separation and divorce. One partner keeps pushing for more sex, and the other partner keeps pulling further away to avoid sex. Resentments and bitterness develop on both sides. Life becomes difficult for both of them as needs are not met, and the currency of love runs out. The opposite side of that coin is that instead of pushing for more, a pervasive indifference and apathy sets into the relationship. Still, no one is happy with this solution either. But mismatched libido doesn't have to be a deal-breaker. Mismatched libido is actually the norm and not the exception, but the degree of mismatch is generally the sticking point. The most common configuration is that the man has a higher sex drive than the woman, but it can be the other way around.

For the longest time, I thought I didn't like sex. Why? Because my husband and I had a mismatch in desire for sex (his was higher), it was a struggle to get in the mood even if I "kinda wanted to," and my husband would flat out tell me "You don't like sex, and I do" whenever we would discuss our sex life. One day after a failed attempt to have sex, I was thinking about what was happening in our bedroom. And I was asking myself, "How can I have more sex if I don't even like sex?" Almost immediately, another question popped into my head. "Do you like sex?" It stopped me dead in my tracks of rumination! "Do I like sex?" I asked myself. The answer initially surprised me.

"Yes!"

And as I thought about it more, I realized that I had always enjoyed sex and remembered being excited for it in the past. I remembered how energized I would get after having sex, feeling like I was on Cloud 9! Yes, I liked sex! I liked the sensations, the closeness and connection, and the afterglow. But my current reality wasn't showing that.

My current reality was that I hardly wanted it, and it was a major struggle to get in the mood even when I did want to do it. So, why was I having problems? My brain had lumped together my struggle to get in the mood with my husband's frequent refrain that I didn't like sex and that equated to dread for sex. This led to me believing that I didn't like sex, even though I did. And that one thing created a negative reality for me, a self-fulfilling prophecy of sorts, but after that day, I was able to address what was happening.

It is time to start asking some questions if your relationship is suffering from a mismatched libido. The first question is what do you want your sex life to be? The next question is are you willing to do the work to make it a reality? Sometimes, the reason for the mismatch is actually due to relationship discord, and that has to be addressed. Sometimes, it can be due to bad habits, like staying up late on your phone and not getting enough sleep. Sometimes, it can be due to fatigue and overwhelming responsibilities. Whatever the reason, it is important to assess what is going on, and then come up with a plan to address it.

The best way to manage this is through communication, managing expectations, and being respectful of each other's wants and needs. However, this is not always easy to do on your own. Getting professional help from a therapist or counselor may be necessary to even start the conversation because these are often emotionally charged conversations. Another thing is to make sure to give each other grace when things don't go as planned. You can agree that you are going to have sex twice a week, but things happen...know that it is not a reflection of the love or lack thereof between the two of you (for the high sex-drive partner).

Notes

Notes

Notes

Notes

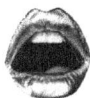

CHAPTER 11

WHAT IS A LIBIDO COACH?

So, what exactly is a libido coach? These days, it requires a little less explanation as life coaching has become more mainstream. My work falls under the umbrella of life coaching, but my focus is more specialized to work with women who are experiencing struggles in their life around sex and desire. A libido coach can help you to develop a different, more positive perspective on what you are experiencing. A libido coach will journey with you on a deep dive to uncover the root of the problem. A libido coach can help you to know what is normal and can help you to create a new normal in the bedroom. A libido coach can guide you in having hard conversations with your partner around sex. A libido coach can transform your life.

What would it mean to your relationship for sex to flow more freely between you and your partner?

What would it mean if the thought of sex didn't make you feel awkward, and you stopped hiding in the bathroom pretending you have some stomach issue, waiting your partner out until they fall asleep, so you don't have to have sex tonight?

What if I told you that the only thing keeping you from a vibrant, passionate, and hot sex life was one word, would you believe me? I mean, who doesn't want a better sex life? Most women that I talk to want a better sex life but don't know how to make it happen. Is that you?

You want more sex? I got you!

You want more orgasms! I got you!

You just want to make sex fun again? I got you!

We tap into the power of the B - spot and brain chemistry, exploring what fires you up and upgrading your life, your love, and your libido.

Who wants to feel more feminine and sexier?

Who wants to increase the connection in their intimate relationship?

Who wants to have more sex and more orgasms?

Notes

Notes

Notes

Notes

THANK YOU

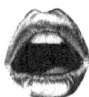

Thank you to all the women who shared their struggles and experiences of dissatisfaction. I am humbled that you entrusted me to witness your vulnerabilities and provide a way to help you untangle the ball of all the things that were blocking you from living your best sex life ever! I am pleased that you now are able to engage in sex without fear, guilt, or dread. I know that you are going out into the world and making positive changes simply because you are spreading the positivity that was poured into you and that you continue to surround yourself with. And not only have you learned about yourself, but you are also changing lives and sharing my legacy with all the girls and women who you come into contact with - showing them what a vibrant, passionate, confident, and sexy woman actually is. You are expanding their vision for what is possible.

Thank you!

DOES THIS SOUND FAMILIAR?

You get home, make dinner, get the kids situated, and then you see your bae making googly eyes at you because they want to get busy tonight. And all you're thinking is, "Not tonight! There is no way I have the energy or the desire for sex tonight!"

If there were a way to quickly flip the script and turn your desire on, would you want to know the secret? As a thank you for purchasing this book, I want to offer you a special gift. Discover the secrets to get out of the daily grind and get in the mood in 15 minutes or less.

- Get expert advice to help you get excited about sex again.
- Connect to your feminine essences easily.
- Learn tips for getting in the mood quickly.
- Stop dreading sex with your partner.

You don't have to continue to suffer, hiding in the bathroom waiting for your partner to go to sleep so that you don't have to say no again.

Go to
www.jumpstartthejumpoff.com
for your FREE video series and Get Your Sexy Back!

ABOUT THE AUTHOR

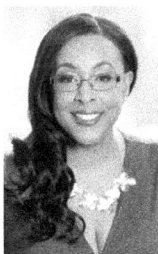

Dr. Brandye Wilson-Manigat, a.k.a. "Dr. Brandye," is among the country's most well-known OB/GYN physicians and surgeons. She is called upon by various local and national media outlets to give a fresh perspective and new information on women's health trends.

She is the founder and chief medical advisor for DrBrandyeMD.com, where she has created a safe space to discuss real-world strategies to help women learn the truth about sex and orgasms, and embrace their feminine essence, so they feel good both inside and outside of the bedroom. She is also the CEO of Women's Libido Institute, which focuses on educating doctors and women's health providers on how to care for women with libido challenges.

Born and raised in South Central Los Angeles, California, Dr. Brandye earned her undergraduate degree from the University of California at Riverside, her doctor of medicine from the David Geffen School of Medicine at UCLA/Charles R. Drew University of Medicine and Science, and completed her residency training at Rochester General Hospital in Rochester, New York.

Learn more at DrBrandyeMD.com

purposely created
P U B L I S H I N G

CREATING DISTINCTIVE BOOKS
WITH INTENTIONAL RESULTS

We're a collaborative group of creative masterminds
with a mission to produce high-quality books to position
you for monumental success in the marketplace.

Our professional team of writers, editors, designers,
and marketing strategists work closely together to ensure
that every detail of your book is a clear representation
of the message in your writing.

Want to know more?
Write to us at info@publishyourgift.com
or call (888) 949-6228

Discover great books, exclusive offers, and more at
www.PublishYourGift.com

Connect with us on social media

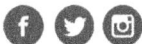

@publishyourgift